Contents

Introduction

Aims of this guide

This guide provides an overview of the evidence that group singing can be beneficial for mental health and wellbeing. We are not concerned with specialised music therapy as a clinical intervention. Such work is undertaken by a suitably qualified and registered music therapist in appropriate clinical settings. Hospital settings are not specifically addressed here. Singing groups can be run in hospital settings of course, but they would require collaboration with hospital staff, and attendance may be variable due to participants' health reasons.

Our concern is to offer information and guidance on setting up singing groups for people living in the community who have experience of a diagnosed mental health condition. These include common conditions such as clinical depression or anxiety, and a wide range of other issues including obsessive-compulsive disorders, psychological addictions, self-harming behaviour and psychosis. Such singing groups may also seek to involve family, friends and carers of people with mental health issues.

The guide draws upon the experience of mental health service users in a number of well-established community singing for mental health groups as well as musicians and music therapists with considerable experience of running such groups. It draws especially upon the experience of musicians and health researchers in the Sidney De Haan Research Centre for Arts and Health in establishing and evaluating a network of singing groups for mental health service users and their supporters, which began in September 2009.

Who is this guide for?

This guide is for anyone interested in setting up, running and evaluating singing groups for the benefit of people with mental health issues living in the community. This includes:

- Health professionals who are interested in supporting the development of evidence-based and effective community activities which can promote mental wellbeing and aid recovery

- Managers of voluntary sector organisations working with people with mental health needs in the community who would like to set up singing groups

- People experiencing mental distress, whether mild or moderate, and those with a history of severe and enduring mental illness who are in recovery and working to manage their lives in the community with support

- Family, relatives and friends of people with a history of mental health issues who are looking for an effective means of engagement and social support for their loved ones

- Experienced community musicians interested in setting up singing for health groups who have not previously worked with people with mental health issues

What this guide offers

Information is provided on evidence from case studies and research projects, and links to further resources training. This is not intended as a practical toolkit, but to guide and inform.

Sidney De Haan
Research Centre for Arts and Health

Singing, Wellbeing and Health: context, evidence and practice

Series Editor: Stephen Clift

The aim of this series is to offer guidance on setting up and running singing groups for people with a range of enduring health issues.

They are based on previous research, the learning from singing for health projects in the UK, and the practical experience of members of the Sidney De Haan Research Centre in establishing and evaluating community singing projects since 2004.

1. Singing and Mental Health – Ian Morrison and Stephen Clift

2. Singing and people with COPD – Ian Morrison and Stephen Clift

3. Singing and people with Dementia – Trish Vella-Burrows

4. Singing and people with Parkinson's – Trish Vella-Burrows and Grenville Hancox

Further resources to supplement this guide can be found online at:

www.canterbury.ac.uk/research/centres/SDHR

For further information on training courses associated with these resources please contact Isobel Salisbury, Sidney De Haan Research Centre for Arts and Health, University Centre Folkestone, Folkestone, Kent CT20 1JG
Email: Isobel.Salisbury@canterbury.ac.uk   Telephone: 01303 220 870

The Sidney De Haan Research Centre for Arts and Health would like to thank everyone who helped with the development of this guide: Jane Bentley, Phoene Cave, Shelly Coyne, Udita Everett, Jean Fraser, Liz Hodgson, Vicki Hume, Liv McLennan, Catherine Pestano, Katie Peters, Jane Petto, Nicola Ramsden, Ken Scott, Janet Stansfeld, Sonia Page, Matthew Shipton, Ann Skingley, Saffron Summerfield, Alan Tavener and Rona Topaz.

Authors: Ian Morrison and Stephen Clift
Published: September 2012

Publisher: Canterbury Christ Church University
ISBN: 9781909067035

Sidney De Haan
Research Centre for Arts and Health

Singing, Wellbeing and Health:
context, evidence and practice

Singing and Mental Health

Ian Morrison and Stephen Clift

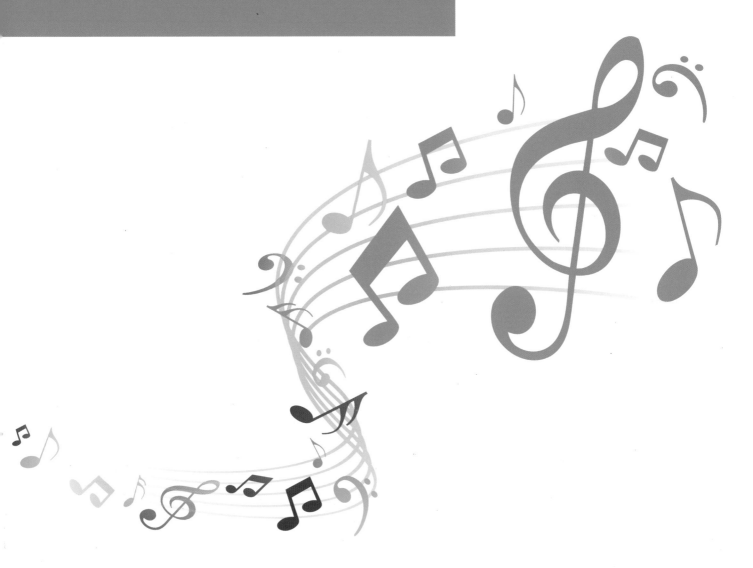

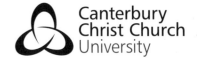
Canterbury
Christ Church
University

Context

The nature and scale of mental health problems in the UK

Mental illness encompasses a spectrum of conditions of varying severity from mild to moderate to severe and enduring. This can range from a temporary stress related absence from work, to a long-term severe mental illness that may have been on-going from childhood, or occurred in teenage to early adulthood. There are many conditions from clinical depression or anxiety, to bipolar affective disorder (manic-depression) and schizophrenia.

The prevalence of mental ill health in the general population is not known exactly. Many cases are probably not reported, possibly due to sufferers not recognising their condition, and so not seeking medical help, or if they do recognise their condition, they do not seek help due to the fear of labelling and stigmatisation. Estimates of 'reported' mental ill health indicated a range of one in six people experiencing the more common mental health problems at any one time, to one in 200 for the severe and enduring problems in a year (Halliwell, Main and Richardson, 2007; See the Mental Health Foundation website for current information on the prevalence of mental health issues: www.mentalhealth.org.uk/help-information/mental-health-statistics).

Patients living in the community may be supported by their GP, or if they need more support, by the secondary mental health services such as a Community Mental Health Team providing a care co-ordinator such as a mental health Occupational Therapist , or a Community Psychiatric Nurse. They will have a Care Programme Approach plan that specifies the clinical support and meaningful activities undertaken, possibly in mental health venues run by mental health third sector voluntary organisations. If a patient relapses, then the patient may be referred to in-patient treatment in hospital psychiatric wards.

The medical model of illness

Psychiatrists and GPs prescribe pharmaceutical drugs to ameliorate the symptoms experienced by patients, with a view to easing the effects of their condition so that they can lead a life within the community. Unfortunately, pharmaceuticals often have side effects. Where significant side effects arise from a drug, psychiatrists and GPs may prescribe other drugs to ameliorate the symptoms experienced by patients. There may be further side effects of these drugs, and so the process continues, which may mean the patient is taking a regimen of several drugs.

It is not a question of the less medication the more healthy a patient is, but more of having what is necessary to function in society with the least discomfort, e.g. a diabetic may need insulin to function, and they would not be healthier by giving up the insulin. Sometimes when patients with mental health issues feel they are improving, they stop taking their medication, with very poor results. The same is true if they forget to take their medication. Some save up their medication for a boost effect, which again can lead to poor results. This is not to be confused with adjustments to dose, as permitted by the prescriber, in order to tailor medication to the needs of the patient. Sometimes patients are having their medication adjusted by a psychiatrist or GP, which can be a difficult time while this takes place, and it can take several months for this to settle down.

Social support in recovery

The medical model of diagnosis, treatment and cure, or management of the condition if cure isn't possible, has been described above in relation to mental ill health. A patient supported by clinical staff and at a stage in their recovery that enables them to live in the community, possibly with the support of third sector mental health voluntary organisations, may be ready to engage in activities which can help them improve their sense of mental wellbeing and re-engagement with others.

Here, the emphasis is on supporting patients' social needs and their gradually increasing empowerment in choice and directing their lives, which includes such issues as education, employment, income, and housing.

From this point of view, mental ill health can be seen as period of profound loss for the patient of the following features of good psychological and social wellbeing:

- Positive feelings
- Expectation and hope
- Self-belief
- Abilities and skills
- Social support and network
- Organisation and structure

People with mental health challenges need support and interventions to help them re-build or develop these aspects of wellbeing. People who actively engage in group singing can benefit in these many different ways.

The salutogenic model of health

A useful model of positive health comes from the perspective of Health Promotion and Antonovsky's salutogenic model of health (Antonovsky, 1987 and 1996). In Antonovsky's model, good health is promoted through 'generalised resistance resources'. It is when resistance resources are inadequate to restore health balance, or manage stress, that an individual breaks down (Antonovsky, 1972). These resistance resources are represented by the concept of 'sense of coherence', which consists of three components: comprehensibility, manageability and meaningfulness (Antonovsky, 1987 and 1993), and these are defined as follows:

Sense of coherence: A global orientation that expresses the extent to which one has a pervasive, enduring though dynamic feeling of confidence that:

- the stimuli deriving from one's internal and external environments in the course of living are structured, predictable, and explicable;
- the resources are available to one to meet the demands posed by the stimuli;
- these demands are challenges, worthy of investment and engagement.

Antonovsky (1987, p19)

Comprehensibility: The person who experiences the world as comprehensible expects that future stimuli will be predictable or, when they do come as surprises, will be orderable and explicable.

Manageability: People who experience their world as manageable have the sense that, aided by their own resources or by those of trustworthy others, they will be able to cope.

Meaningfulness: A person who experiences the world as meaningful will not be overcome by unhappy experiences but will experience them as challenges, be determined to seek meaning in them, and do his/her best to overcome them with dignity.

Carstens and Spangenberg (1997, p1212)

For an example of a project designed on the basis of salutogenic principles to support mental health service users into a further education college, see Morrison and Clift, 2006 and Morrison, Stosz and Clift, 2008. For a recent review of Salutogenesis, see Lindstrom and Eriksson, 2010.

The current national policy framework for mental health

The Department of Health published a new cross-government strategy for mental health in 2011 – 'No Health without Mental Health' (Department of Health, 2011). This provides a framework for efforts to improve mental health and wellbeing in the wider population and services for mental health difficulties across the lifespan. The strategy has six ambitious objectives:

- More people will have a positive experience of care and support
- More people with mental health problems will recover
- More people will have good mental health
- Fewer people will experience stigma and discrimination
- Fewer people will suffer avoidable harm
- More people with mental health problems will have good physical health

While the NHS has a key role in achieving these objectives, it cannot do so alone, and effective partnerships between mental health services, local government and charitable and voluntary organisations are essential. The argument of this guide is that community opportunities for people to come together and sing could make a considerable contribution to achieving these objectives – as could many other forms of creative activity and cultural participation. However, singing can be undertaken by almost everybody, even sitting down; all that is needed is to be able to speak, and hear (to be tuneful).

When people with a history of mental illness come together to sing guided by a sensitive and skilled facilitator, they are taking part in an activity which is inherently caring and supportive. Members of choirs get to know one another, form friendships and offer support for one another. For these reasons alone, the experience can contribute to the process of recovery, but in addition there are inherent features of singing and learning new material which helps to promote a sense of wellbeing. Not least is the enjoyment and fun associated with singing; the concentration and sense of achievement that comes from learning something new; the sense of working together in a team cooperatively, and finally the beauty of the final result in performance.

Singing together reflects in fact, all five of the Five Ways to Wellbeing devised by the New Economics Foundation Wellbeing Programme, which the 'No Health without Mental Health' strategy endorses:

- Connect - with people around you
- Be active – walk, run, cycle, dance
- Take notice – catch sight of the beautiful, savour the moment
- Keep learning – makes you more confident as well as being fun
- Give – do something nice for a friend or a stranger

How group singing can help promote mental wellbeing

Group singing can help to address all of the social needs identified above of patients living in the community, with support, and ready to engage socially.

Positive feelings: Singing has been shown to be a joyful and uplifting experience. It generates a sense of positive mood, happiness and enjoyment. Such positive feelings also counteract feelings of stress or anxiety and help to distract people from internal negative thoughts and feelings.

Expectation and hope: Enjoyable activities such as singing with others are things people will look forward to each week. They can become highlights of the week and positive memories remain alive for hours and days afterwards. Where an activity involves working towards a goal such as a performance, there are enhanced expectations of rewarding outcomes.

Self-belief: A change of identity can occur for people with mental health issues by participating in group singing, from thinking of themselves as choir members, rather than patients. This can raise a sense of self-esteem and confidence and performance events can bring a sense of social recognition and status. Performances help to reduce stigma and labelling by others.

Abilities and skills: Confidence is brought about by the ability to repeat previously learned tasks or skills (including social skills), with a high degree of accuracy. Successful skills might also help to improve success in new, related skills, when tried for the first time. Learning new songs or harmonising parts of songs, can help concentration and focus, and stimulate learning and memory. Concentration can also provide a distraction from other concerns, leading to respite from them.

Social support and networking: Singing in a group offers the opportunity to build social capital, encourage social inclusion and raised status of the members, and creates an opportunity for communities to come together.

Organisation and structure: Structure is something that is easily lost when ill. Patients can feel adrift and disconnected. Having the purpose and goal of attending a weekly group can be motivating and create an anchor upon which other weekly activities might build.

Evidence

Case studies

Case studies provide the most abundant evidence of the value of group singing for mental wellbeing. Across the UK, many singing groups have been established for people affected by mental health challenges. A number have run for several years and have proved their value in practice. People with a history of mental health issues would not continue attending singing groups if they didn't derive substantial benefits from the experience. We give here three short case studies based on a fuller account that appears in Clift, Morrison, Vella-Burrows et al. (2011). Each of these was written by people directly involved in setting up the choirs, including mental health service users.

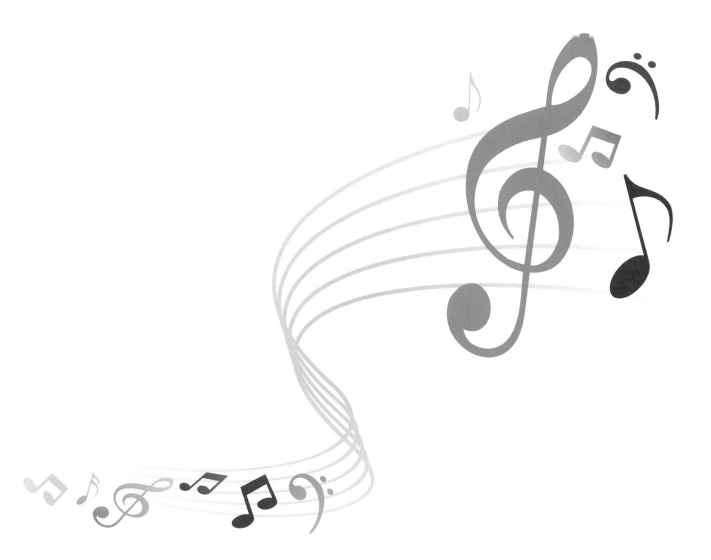

Sing Your Heart Out (Norwich/Norfolk)

Sing Your Heart Out (SYHO) groups meet weekly for singing workshops which are open to mental health service users and supporters, led by Chrissy Parsons-West. The groups meet in several venues across Norfolk and excellent films of SYHO sessions can be viewed on their website (see Resources section). The workshops involve singing in harmony, using rounds, part-songs and simple arrangements from as many styles as possible in order to appeal to a wide range of tastes in music. The songs include easy African songs, spirituals, traditional rounds and arrangements of pop classics. The inclusion of staff, carers, friends, family and anyone from the local community alongside mental service users is one of the key factors in the project's value in combating stigma and facilitating re-integration into ordinary life, especially for service users who have spent time in isolation or in institutional care.

While some people attend very regularly, for others, having to make an ongoing commitment would be a deterrent. For this reason every group is run as an open session and everyone is welcome to drop-in and out as suits them. Choosing repertoire with many potential layers is very helpful, so that each time a song is revisited there is the chance to teach the best-known parts to newcomers while offering new variations to those who have already sung the song many times.

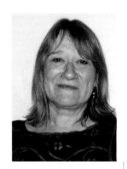

"SYHO is the most interesting and varied teaching project I've ever worked on and also one of the most rewarding. While there have been great moments of musical breakthroughs, the most powerful moments for me have been the 'firsts' which have been brought about through the singing, even if they were not actually being part of the singing! The first time someone's lips have moved to begin to whisper the words of a song – the first time someone lifted her head to make eye contact – the first time someone managed to stay in the room for the whole session, and, most movingly, the first time someone felt that what he sang 'mattered'."

Chrissy Parsons-West
Director of Sing Your Heart Out

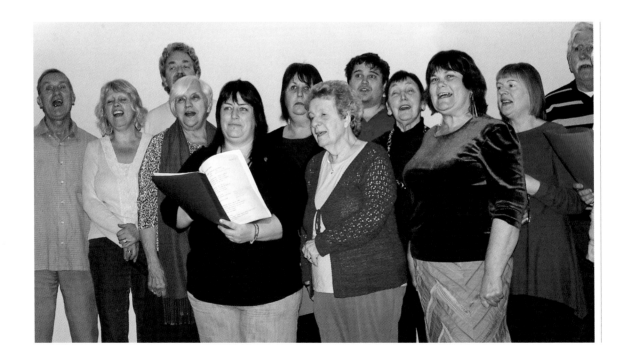

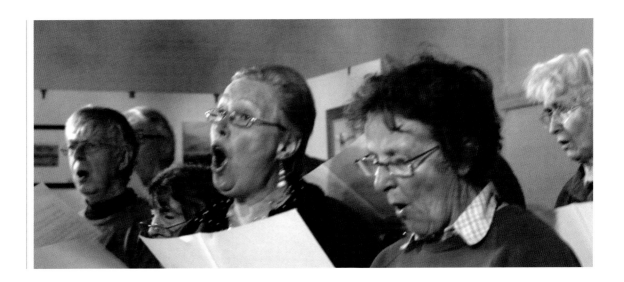

Michaelhouse Chorale, Arts and Minds (Cambridge)

The Michaelhouse Chorale is a choir for mental health service users of any age together with their carers and friends. It was established in November 2007 by the charity Arts and Minds and is run by Sam Hayes. Sessions start with physical and vocal exercises to aid relaxation, and an element of movement and drama is encouraged in some pieces. Percussion is used where appropriate. The songs reflect the taste and capabilities of the participants as some have considerable musical ability and are able to read music, whereas others have never sung before, or not since schooldays. The repertoire ranges from the classical tradition of the mediaeval period - secular and sacred - through to the present day, and popular music. The standard of singing is high, and many pieces feature the elements of singing in harmony, or antiphonally.

The Chorale runs as a 'drop-in', so the number of participants varies from week to week, but can reach 20. The core membership of 14 mental health service users, their carers and others, ranges in age from the early 20s to early 80s. Illnesses include panic attacks, mild and severe clinical depression, bi-polar, schizophrenia, dementia and learning disability. The members were recently asked to choose which of the many pieces they have sung they most enjoy, and what they mean to them. This presented quite a challenge because they all said how much they enjoy everything they sing, whether sacred or secular. They described singing as very important to them, bringing a sense of fellowship and community which is especially helpful and supportive for some members who said they had previously been hiding themselves away as a result of their mental illness.

"My own enjoyment of the weekly sessions has grown, and the opportunity to sing with the members has also reinforced and improved my own singing technique. Having had no previous experience of working with people with a mental health condition I have now read widely around the subject of music – particularly singing – and health. I believe that running the Chorale has had just as much of a positive effect on my own mental wellbeing as it clearly has on the members of the group. I cannot remember a session since the Chorale's foundation when I have not left buoyant and cheerful, and I believe this has a very positive effect on my other conducting work."

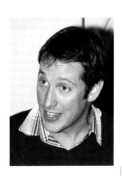

Sam Hayes
Chorale Music Director, Michaelhouse Chorale, Arts and Minds

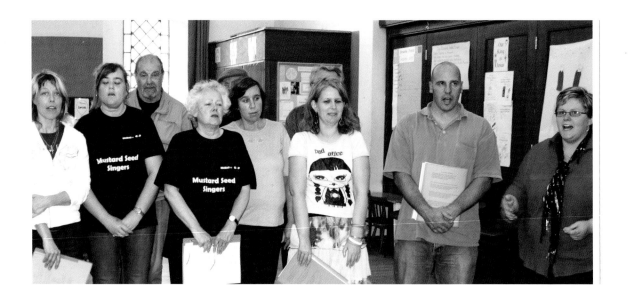

The Mustard Seed Singers (Canterbury)

The Mustard Seed Singers was established by Elle Caldon, herself a mental health service user, to rehearse carols for a Christmas event at the Mustard Seed day centre in Canterbury. Members of the group enjoyed the experience of meeting to sing and then perform so much that they wanted the choir to continue. During 2008, the choir's confidence developed considerably and several public performance events took place, with positive audience reactions which gave the choir great pleasure and a sense of recognition. They have performed regularly since then in many different local venues The choir has a regularly attending core membership of approximately 12-15 people. Most are mental health service users, but the choir also includes partners and friends, family members, together with mental health service professionals.

The repertoire sung by the Mustard Seed Singers is very wide, and includes traditional folk songs, songs from musicals, pop songs, African songs, Gospel songs, and seasonal songs (Christmas carols). All songs are taught by ear, and are unaccompanied. Some are sung in unison, but most have two or more parts. A number of songs have emerged as particular favourites of the group, and these are sung with the greatest vigour and feeling. Members of the choir have sometimes spontaneously expressed their feelings after singing these songs and have reported 'tingling sensations' down the back of the neck, and an enhanced sense of group feeling. During one meeting of the choir, a member arrived a little late looking distressed. In the interval, another member listened to her share details of her day. She said 'I almost didn't come, but I'm glad now I made the effort.' He replied, 'I'm glad you made it. Singing is the best anti-depressant I've ever had!'

"Emotionally people turn up in all sorts of situations and states and sometimes singing can help to calm things down a bit and you've got a focus on something else. I mean physically it helps with breathing and if you have panic attacks, that kind of thing, it all helps and mentally and cognitively it is just a very, very beneficial thing to do. So many people I have spoken to say 'I can't sing' and it's just such a classic that they have been told in childhood or at school or something, and I would just like to challenge that belief because actually most, or probably all people can sing more or less tunefully and it's just an equal playing field, and just give it a go."

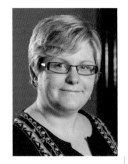

Elle Caldon
Founder and Director of the Mustard Seed Singers

Research evidence on singing and mental health

A systematic review of research on singing and wellbeing (Clift, Nicol, Raisbeck et al., 2010) has revealed a relatively small and varied corpus of research. Of the studies reviewed, a number stand out as particularly relevant to the question of whether group singing has a potential role in aiding the recovery and social inclusion of people with mental health needs.

Bailey and Davidson (2002) have shown considerable wellbeing benefits from choral singing for a small sample of homeless men and replicated these findings in further studies of singers in choirs in disadvantaged and privileged communities. Two quasi-experimental studies have also reported positive health impacts from group singing for elderly people using standardised measures and objective indicators of wellbeing and health. Houston, McKee, Carroll et al. (1998) report improvements in levels of anxiety and depression in nursing home residents, following a four-week programme of singing, and Cohen, Perlstein, Chapline et al. (2006) found improvements in both mental and physical health in a group of elderly people participating in a community choir for one year.

Clift, Hancox, Morrison et al. (2010) report the largest study on choral singing and wellbeing undertaken to date. Their cross-national survey took the World Health Organisation's definition of health as a starting point and utilised the short form of the WHO Quality of Life questionnaire (WHOQOL-BREF) to gather data on 1124 choral singers drawn from choirs in Australia, England and Germany. In addition, singers completed a specially constructed 12-item 'effects of choral singing scale' and gave written accounts of the effects of choral singing on wellbeing and health in response to open questions.

Clift, Hancox, Morrison et al. (2010) and Clift and Hancox (2010) examined written accounts of the effects of choral singing on wellbeing given by participants with relatively low psychological wellbeing as assessed by the WHOQOL-BREF, and high scores on the singing scale indicating a strong perceived impact of singing on a sense of personal well-being. Four categories of significant personal and health challenges were disclosed by members of this group: enduring mental health problems; family/relationship problems; physical health challenges and recent bereavement, and in all cases, singing provided support in coping with such challenges. Written comments from members of choirs reporting these challenges show clearly the power of singing in promoting mental wellbeing.

In 2009, the Sidney De Haan Research Centre for Arts and Health established a network of singing groups for mental health service users in towns across East Kent. The evaluation conducted during the first year of this project has provided powerful evidence of the value of singing groups for promoting recovery and maintaining wellbeing among people with a history of enduring mental health challenges (Clift and Morrison, 2011).

The East Kent Singing for Mental Health Network

The idea for this project developed from links between the Sidney De Haan Centre and the Mustard Seed Singers, a choir established in Canterbury by Elle Caldon in 2007. Seven new singing groups were established in towns across East Kent (Sheerness, Faversham, Whitstable, Broadstairs, Deal, Folkestone and Ashford) during September 2009. The choirs are supported by a team of five facilitators. The project has continued for a second year and currently, a total of approximately 150 participants are involved in the network.

During the first year, choirs met weekly over three terms of 11-12 weeks. At the end of each term members of the choirs were asked to complete a questionnaire called 'Clinical Outcomes in Routine Evaluation' (CORE). This instrument is widely used across the UK in the on-going evaluation of counselling and therapy provision for people with mental health issues. In addition, qualitative evaluation took place through observation and verbal and written feedback from participants (including health professionals) and facilitators.

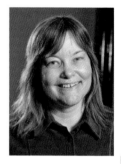

"Some of the research carried out with the choirs across East Kent have used tools to actually measure how people feel after they sing as opposed to how they were before they sung; how they felt across time as well, so how being involved in the choir for several weeks or months has impacted on their improved wellbeing and mental health recovery and confidence and, all the things that go with being involved in these choirs. So it's actually being able to capture those outcomes and demonstrate those outcomes and that is what is so crucial to what the research project is about. It's just life changing for some people. I've actually seen some people's lives drastically changed by being involved in the choirs, especially people who have had long term mental illness who are involved in these choirs has been amazing with the actual results we have seen so far."

Jill Knight
Occupational Therapist, Kent and Medway
NHS and Social Care Partnership Trust

Findings from the CORE questionnaire

The CORE questionnaire consists of 34 items which people respond to on a five point scale (0-4). Sets of these items form scales of wellbeing, psychological problems, functioning in daily life and risk behaviours and the score is the mean rating on each scale. The higher the mean score a person gains on these scales the greater the degree of mental and social difficulties they are reporting, and any mean above 1 indicates a clinically significant level of difficulty. The following graph (Figure 1), based on 26 members of the network who enrolled at the start of the project and attended consistently, shows the change in CORE scale scores over a period of eight months. Few members of the group were reporting 'risk' behaviours or feelings (e.g. suicidal thoughts, attempts at self-harm), but means on the wellbeing, problems and functioning scales were all above the clinical significant level at end of the first term of the project, and then fell consistently over the period of eight months. All of these changes are highly statistically significant.

Figure 1: Changes in COREOM sub-scales over three terms (N=26)

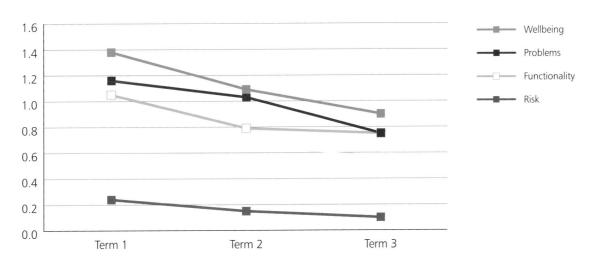

Qualitative feedback from participants indicated even more graphically the positive changes experienced over this period:

> I have bipolar disorder. When I am depressed, singing in the group and coming together with other people lifts my mood and gives me something positive and productive to focus on. When I am manic, singing is something I can channel my extra energy into and express my enthusiasm for life through. The choir provides structure and purpose in an otherwise sometimes empty life.

> It helps me to structure my week, to have something to keep going for. I enjoy meeting all types of people. It has been very good to meet new people who have experiences similar to my own. If I feel I might have a panic attack, I know how to breathe properly which helps. I would have very little reason to leave the house if it wasn't doing choirs.

> Music is a very important therapeutic and enjoyment factor in my life. The singing group has meant that I have been actively involved for once rather than in the audience and it's been a valuable experience. I find any group situation hard and testing. To share and experience music with a group has enabled me to overcome some of the barriers I would usually feel. I have managed to attend singing on several occasions when feeling extremely stressed. I found to my surprise and delight that it did indeed not only provide a distraction but transformed my mood. I have been reminded that I am often my own worst enemy and refuse to do things through fear of failure.

Public performances

An important feature of this project is that singing groups are part of a network, each learning and rehearsing the same core repertoire of material. This has made it possible to bring the choirs together for larger choral performance events, and there have been three such events during 2010-2011 (the photograph below shows the choirs performing at the Granville Theatre Ramsgate in June 2010. See the Resources section of this guide for details of a film of this event).

Such performances demonstrate the power of singing to bring people together and support recovery from mental ill-health; they promote social inclusion, social capital and normalization for people with mental health issues, and serve to challenge misconceptions, stigma and prejudice associated with mental illness.

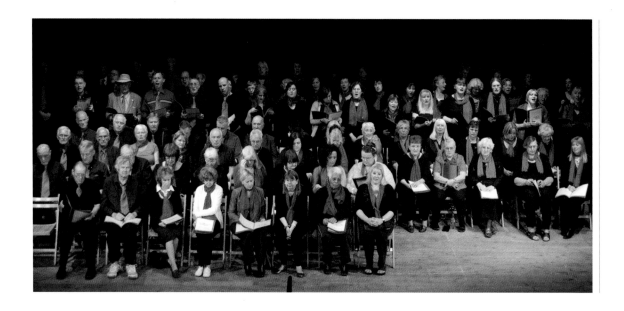

Practice

Guidance on setting up and running singing groups for mental health

The facilitator

The role of the facilitator is key in any musical group, and especially so in amateur choirs. The facilitator needs to be musically skilled but equally socially skilled and sensitive to the needs, circumstances and capacities of the people they are working with in a singing group. Musicians with experience of leading choirs, who are interested in working with people with a history of mental health difficulties, may feel in need of training. A good way forward would be to contact organisations and projects with experience in this area to arrange a visit and explore possibilities for mentoring or training. Some ideas are given in the resource section of this guide.

The repertoire

A singing group for people with mental health needs is concerned first and foremost with meeting the psychological and social needs of the people involved. Therefore it is important for the range of music and songs to be wide to appeal to varied musical tastes in any group.

Many of the participants will be inexperienced singers. As the participants are mainly interested in health, the repertoire needs to be interesting even if sung in unison, but be capable of gradually increasing the challenge over time by adding rounds (canons), and simple but effective harmonies. All of this should be achieved without stressing participants, which could negatively affect them. For the participants it is about the joy and happiness of singing, rather than tackling complicated or difficult tasks. For this to be enjoyable, it is necessary to produce a quality that they are prepared to perform in public to their peers, friends, and relatives, which brings the added benefits of social inclusion, being valued, giving back, status etc. Obviously it's good to reach the best level they are capable of, but not at the expense of their health. It is primarily about the participants' requirements, not the aspirations of the singing group leader. Another consideration is that if new people join an existing singing group, there need to be parts that new inexperienced participants can easily slot into and feel part of the group straight away. Otherwise they will feel uncomfortable and may not return.

The experience of the singing for mental health groups featured in our case studies are of interest. In each of them, a varied repertoire has been sung by the group, but different songs have become particular favourites and generally express some sentiments of significance for the group and its members. This illustrates the point that often it is not just the music that is important in singing, but also the lyrics.

The repertoire sung by the Mustard Seed Singers, for example, is very wide, and in the main has been chosen by the leader, but some songs have been requested by members. It includes traditional folk songs (e.g. *What shall we do with the drunken sailor?*), songs from musicals (e.g. *Ascot gavotte* from *My Fair Lady*), pop songs (e.g. a Beatles medley), African songs (e.g. *Sen wa de dende*), Gospel songs (e.g. *As I went down to the river to pray*) and seasonal songs (Christmas carols). Songs have gradually been added to the group's song book, which now contains over 30 songs, many of which have been sung repeatedly in rehearsals and performed in public. All songs are taught by ear, and are unaccompanied. Some are sung in unison, but most have two or more parts. A number of the songs are sung as canons.

The songs are interesting musically for the quality of their sound, but also for their lyrics, which address social and psychological challenges, which anyone might face in their lives, and three examples can be given to illustrate these ideas. The first of these '*I got rhythm*' (George and Ira Gershwin), is uplifting and energetic and is accompanied with finger clicking and thigh slapping! Individuals have literally 'got rhythm' and have 'got music' flowing through their bodies. The song also refers to the importance of having loving support, having dreams and a positive outlook on life.

The following passage is particularly moving when sung by a group of people who have had more than their fair share of troubles:

> *Old man trouble*
> *I don't mind him*
> *You won't find him 'round my door*
> *I got starlight*
> *I got sweet dreams*
> *I got my man (love)*
> *Who could ask for anything more?*

A second song that is affecting in a different way is '*Lean on me*' (Bill Whithers). It speaks not only of the need for friendship and support in the face of adversity, but recognises that everyone at some time in their life needs someone to lean on:

> *Lean on me, when you're not strong*
> *And I'll be your friend*
> *I'll help you carry on*
> *For it won't be long*
> *'Til I'm gonna need*
> *Somebody to lean on*

In a choir made up of mental health service users and professional workers, this gives a particularly powerful message in the context of mental health care. People facing challenges to their mental health are looking first and foremost for personal and professional friends they can rely upon to help get them through their difficulties, and this can be as true for professionals in health services as anyone else.

The third song, which is perhaps the signature tune of the choir, is '*The Rose*' (Bette Midler) – a song with harmonies almost certain to create chill experiences in performers and listeners alike, and which can readily bring tears to the eyes. The song speaks of 'love' and the ways in which the complications of love in its many forms, including addictions and dependencies, can be damaging in our lives. But essentially the song is about hope and self-belief. Belief that all of us can find within ourselves the resources and sense of self-worth central to a capacity for resilience in the face of life's challenges:

> *When the night has been too lonely*
> *And the road has been too long*
> *And you think that love is only*
> *For the lucky and the strong*
> *Just remember, in the winter*
> *Far beneath the bitter snows*
> *Lies the seed that with the sun's love*
> *In the spring, becomes the rose*

Guidance on monitoring and evaluation

In setting up a new singing group for people with mental health needs it is important to consider the issue of monitoring and evaluation from the outset. Indeed if a group is funded by a statutory or voluntary body, some processes of evaluation and regular reports may be required.

Gathering evidence on the process and outcomes of any project which aims to improve wellbeing and health is also essential to check whether the activity is having the desired effects.

Evaluation can be challenging and time-consuming to do well, and where possible the assistance of an external evaluator is ideal – not least because it gives some assurance of the independence and objectivity of the evidence gathered.

There are many approaches to evaluation, some simple and others more complex, and a wide range of techniques of information gathering and processing can be followed. Reference to previously published research described earlier in this guide can be useful in appreciating the range of approaches that have been adopted. For simplicity, however, here are three possibilities of increasing complexity:

Qualitative monitoring of process and outcomes

The simplest approach is to gather comments from participants on their experiences during the singing sessions and what they feel they have gained from their involvement. Simple questionnaires can be used for this purpose with some structured questions, but also space for people to write their own comments. The quotations given in the account of the East Kent 'Singing for Health' Network project above were gathered in just this way – by asking people to write open-ended accounts of their experiences in their singing groups.

Use of structured pre-validated questionnaires

A further step is to attempt to measure outcomes from participation in the singing groups using previously published questionnaires which are the result of a rigorous process of development and validation to show that they give meaningful results. Two simple and freely available questionnaires are worth considering in evaluating a new group: the short form of the Warwick Edinburgh Mental Wellbeing Scale, and the short form of the Clinical Outcomes in Routine Evaluation questionnaire (CORE). These questionnaires would take no more than 10 minutes for participants to complete, and so they make very little demand on people. If participants are asked to complete them before the start of a singing group and then at intervals, it will be possible to see whether any improvements are taking place.

Controlled experiments on the effects of singing

The second approach to evaluation has the merit of attempting to measure change with a validated questionnaire. It has the obvious weakness however that the changes observed could have happened anyway or as a result of many other influences in people's lives in addition to being part of a choir. For this reason, some kind of 'control' group is often recommended in evaluations of any project to provide a point of comparison. In the ideal situation, such control groups would be established at the same time as the singing group and participants would be randomly assigned to the singing group and a control (either no intervention or some form of alternative activity). Skingley, Clift, Coulton and Rodriguez (2011) present a protocol for such a study, which aimed to assess the effects of group singing on the mental wellbeing of people aged 60+. Randomised controlled trials or RCTs as they called, are extremely costly and time-consuming and also difficult to set up. Nevertheless, if any form of comparison group can be included in an evaluation it is likely to strengthen the study. For example, people with mental health issues in a singing group could be compared with a similar group of people involved in a different group activity (a gardening, painting or reading group for example). Another approach would be to follow a group of people over several months before they start to sing, and compare what they say about their mental wellbeing during that period with their experience once the singing group starts.

Research ethics

Where a singing for mental health group is operating in a community and participants refer themselves, and the group facilitator is keen to gather feedback, formal ethical approval would not be needed. It would still be important that information is gathered in accordance with sound ethical principles (e.g. informed consent and care over confidentiality and data protection). Where an external evaluator is involved they will need to seek ethical approval from an appropriate body (e.g. university researchers would gain ethical approval from an ethics committee in their institution). Where evaluation is undertaken it is important to publish the findings. This not only furthers the field, but also supports future funding applications. If you wish to publish in professional or peer reviewed journals, they will almost certainly require evidence that the study has been through ethical approval.

Sources of support and funding

There is increasing interest across the UK in the idea that singing can be beneficial for mental wellbeing for everyone, and especially for people who may be troubled with recurrent or enduring problems with mental health. Organisations and individuals with experience in this area are available to give help and support to anyone interested in setting up new groups, and details can be found in the resources section in this guide.

Funding is a perennial challenge, although the costs involved in setting up and running a group are not very great. Funds are needed for the facilitator's fee (and perhaps an accompanist or a system to play backing tracks), a venue and song sheets. Musicians should work with local mental health charities and support services to discuss practical possibilities and sources of support, and local NHS mental health trusts and local commissioning consortia can be approached to explore sources of funding. For more ambitious projects, funders such as the Big Lottery and other charities with an interest in the arts could be approached.

The voluntary organisation Funding Buddies, is currently able to offer help with identifying sources of funding and a mentor scheme for bid-writing. They also offer a written toolkit (for Kent see **www.fundingbuddiesinkent.org.uk**)

With the introduction of personalised budgets for health and social care, this may also be a source of funding for singing for health groups, if participants, individually or collectively, choose to use some of their budget to pay for such an activity.

Resources

Major mental health charities

Mental Health Foundation: The Mental Health Foundation is the UK's leading mental health research, policy and service improvement charity. They are committed to reducing the suffering caused by mental ill health and to help people lead mentally healthier lives. They help people to survive, recover from and prevent mental health problems. Excellent source of information about the nature and scale of mental health issues in the UK, and mental health policy. **www.mentalhealth.org.uk**

MIND: Mind helps people take control of their mental health. They do this by providing high-quality information and advice, and campaigning to promote and protect good mental health for everyone. They can also provide information about local MIND centres across the country, which provide support for people with mental health challenges and their families. **www.mind.org.uk**

Rethink: Rethink provide services, information and support to make a practical and positive difference to people with severe mental illness and their families. They can provide information about support services available across the country. **www.rethink.org**

Singing for mental wellbeing projects

East Kent 'Singing for Health' Network Project: This project involves a network of eight singing groups across East Kent for mental health service users. It was set up in September 2009 by the Sidney De Haan Research Centre for Arts and Health. In June 2010, the singing groups came together at The Granville Theatre, Ramsgate to give a public performance. For a short film about the project see. **www.youtube.com/watch?v=Mlsoii8px04**

Sing For Your Life: A registered charity established in 2005 to improve quality of life, health and wellbeing for older people through participation in musical activities. The core activity of Sing For Your Life is a network of Silver Song Clubs, regular sessions of social and community music making for older people. There are now over 30 Silver Song Clubs meeting across the South East of England. **www.singforyourlife.org.uk**

Sing Your Heart Out: Sing Your Heart Out is a series of singing workshops designed to get people together to enjoy themselves, and to gain the known benefits to mental health from singing. The workshops are open to anyone who is a present or past user of Norfolk mental health services, their family, friends, carers, any support workers, and staff or anyone interested. **www.syho.org**

Music organisations for support and training

Natural Voice Practitioners Network: The Natural Voice Practitioners' Network is an organisation for Practitioners who share a common ethos and approach to voice work. NVPN believes that singing is everyone's birthright and they are committed to teaching styles that are accepting and inclusive of all, regardless of musical experience and ability. **www.naturalvoice.net**

Nordoff Robbins: Nordoff Robbins is a national charity that focuses on music therapy to support the lives of children and adults across the UK. The organisation also provides one-off or short programmes on developing musical skills and help with working with community groups. **www.nordoff-robbins.org.uk**

Sense of Sound: Sense of Sound's mission is to always be at the forefront of vocal education and to provide training, employment and promotional opportunities at the highest level in the creative industries for singers and songwriters across the UK and internationally. Sense of Sound delivers high-quality inclusive vocal training, develops and nurtures aspiring singers. **www.senseofsound.org**

Sound Sense: Sound Sense is a membership organisation that provides support to organisations and individuals who help people make music in their communities through leading music workshops and teaching. **www.soundsense.org**

References

Antonovsky, A. (1972) Breakdown: A needed fourth step in the conceptual armamentarium of modern medicine. Social Science and Medicine, 6, 537-544

Antonovsky, A. (1987) Unravelling the Mystery of Health. How People Manage Stress and Stay Well. San Francisco, Jossey-Bass Inc.

Antonovsky, A. (1993) The structure and properties of the sense of coherence scale. Social Science and Medicine, 36, 6, 725-733.

Antonovsky, A. (1996) The salutogenic model as a theory to guide health promotion. Health Promotion International, 11, 1, 11-18.

Bailey, B.A. and Davidson, J.W. (2002) Adaptive characteristics of group singing: perceptions from members of a choir for homeless men, Musicae Scientiae, VI, 2, 221-256.

Bailey, B.A. and Davidson, J.W. (2005). Effects of group singing and performance for marginalized and middle-class singers, Psychology of Music, 33, 3, 269-303.

Bengel, J. Strittmatter, R. and Willmann, H. (1999) What Keeps People Healthy? – The Current State of Discussion and the Relevance of Antonovsky's Salutogenic Model of Health – Vol 4. Germany, Federal Centre for Health Education.

Carstens, J. A. and Spangenberg, J. J. (1997) Major depression: A breakdown in sense of coherence? Psychological Reports, 80, 1211-1220.

Clift, S. and Hancox, G. (2001) The perceived benefits of singing: findings from preliminary surveys with a university college choral society. Journal of the Royal Society for the Promotion of Health, 121, 4, 248-256.

Clift, S. and Hancox, G. (2010) The significance of choral singing for sustaining psychological wellbeing: Findings from a survey of choristers in England, Australia and Germany, Music Performance Research, 3, 1, 79-96. Available at: http://mpr-online.net

Clift, S. and Morrison, I. (2011) Group singing fosters mental health and wellbeing: Findings from the East Kent 'Singing for Health' Network Project, Mental Health and Social Inclusion, 15, 2, 88-97.

Clift, S., Hancox, G., Morrison, I., Hess, B., Kreutz, G. and Stewart, D. (2010) Choral singing and psychological wellbeing: Quantitative and qualitative findings from English choirs in a cross-national survey, Journal of Applied Arts and Health, 1, 1, 19-34.

Clift, S. M., Hancox, G., Staricoff, R., Whitmore, C., with Morrison, I. and Raisbeck, M. (2008), 'Singing and Health: A Systematic Mapping and Review of Non-Clinical Studies', Canterbury: Canterbury Christ Church University. Available at: www.canterbury.ac.uk/research/centres/SDHR

Clift, S., Morrison, I., Vella-Burrows, T., Hancox, G., Caldon, E., Perry, U., Holden, P., Parsons-West, C., Hesketh Moore, K., Rowland-Jones, C. and Hayes, S. (2011) Singing for mental health and wellbeing: Community initiatives in England, In Brader, A. (Ed.) Songs of Resilience, Cambridge: Cambridge Scholars Press.

Clift, S., Nicol, J., Raisbeck, M., Whitmore, C. and Morrison, I. (2011) Group singing, wellbeing and health: A systematic mapping of research evidence, The UNESCO Journal, 2, 1. Available at: www.abp.unimelb.edu.au/unesco/ejournal

Cohen, G.D., Perlstein, S., Chapline, J., Kelly, J., Firth, K.M. and Simmens, S. (2006). The impact of professionally conducted cultural programs on the physical health, mental health, and social functioning of older adults, The Gerontologist, 46, 6, 726-734.

Department of Health (2011) No Health without Mental Health: A cross-government mental health outcomes strategy for people of all ages London: HM Stationery Office.

Halliwell, E., Main, L. and Richardson, C. (2007) The Fundamental Facts: The latest facts and figures on mental health London: Mental Health Foundation.

Houston, D.M., McKee, K.J., Carroll, L. and Marsh, H. (1998). Using humour to promote psychological wellbeing in residential homes for older people, Aging and Mental Health, 2, 4, 328-332.

Lindstrom, B. and Eriksson, M. (2010) The Hitchhiker's Guide to Salutogenesis, Salutogenic Pathways to Health Promotion. Helsinki: IUHPE.

Morrison, I. and Clift, S. M. (2006) Mental health promotion through supported further education: The value of Antonovsky's salutogenic model of health, Health Education, 106, 5, 365-380.

Morrison, I, Stosz, L. M. and Clift, S.M (2008) An evidence base for mental health promotion through supported education – A practical application of Antonovsky's salutogenic model of health. International Journal of Health Promotion and Education, 46, 1, 11-20.

Skingley, A., Clift, S. M., Coulton, S.P., and Rodriguez, J. (2011) The effectiveness and cost-effectiveness of a participative community singing programme as a health promotion initiative for older people: Protocol for a randomised controlled trial, BMC Public Health, 11, 142. Available at: www.biomedcentral.com/content/pdf/1471-2458-11-142.pdf